i love apples

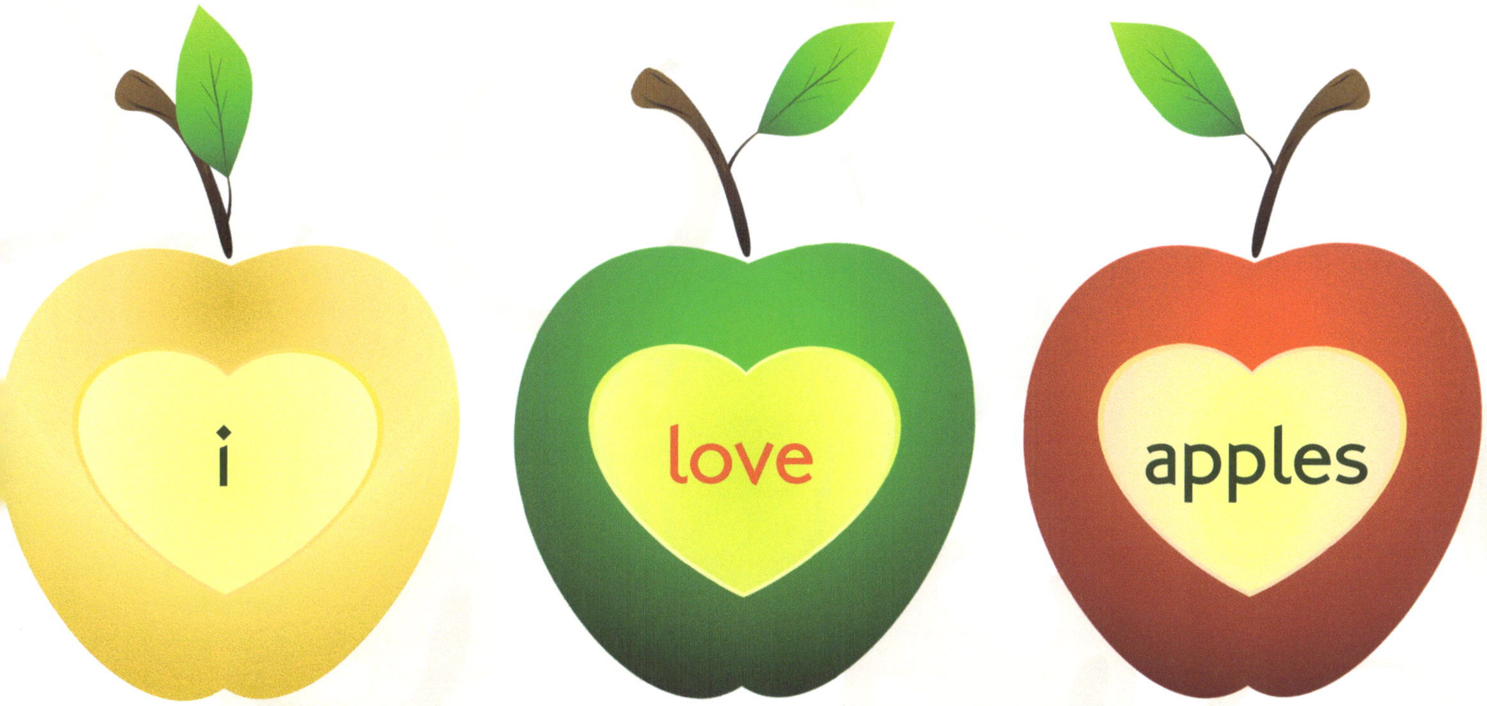

By Tim Dailey
Illustrated by Ian Lusung

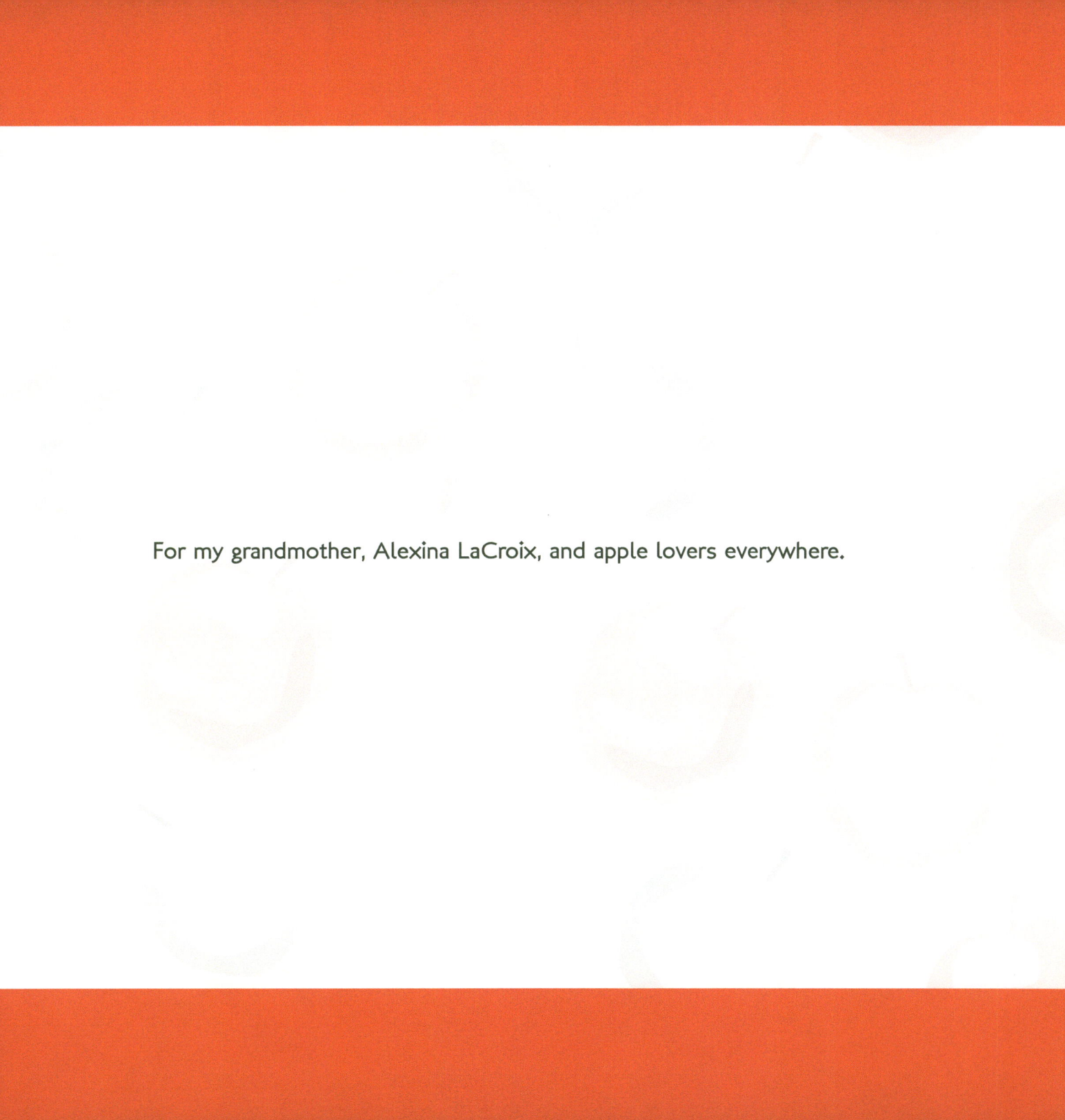

For my grandmother, Alexina LaCroix, and apple lovers everywhere.

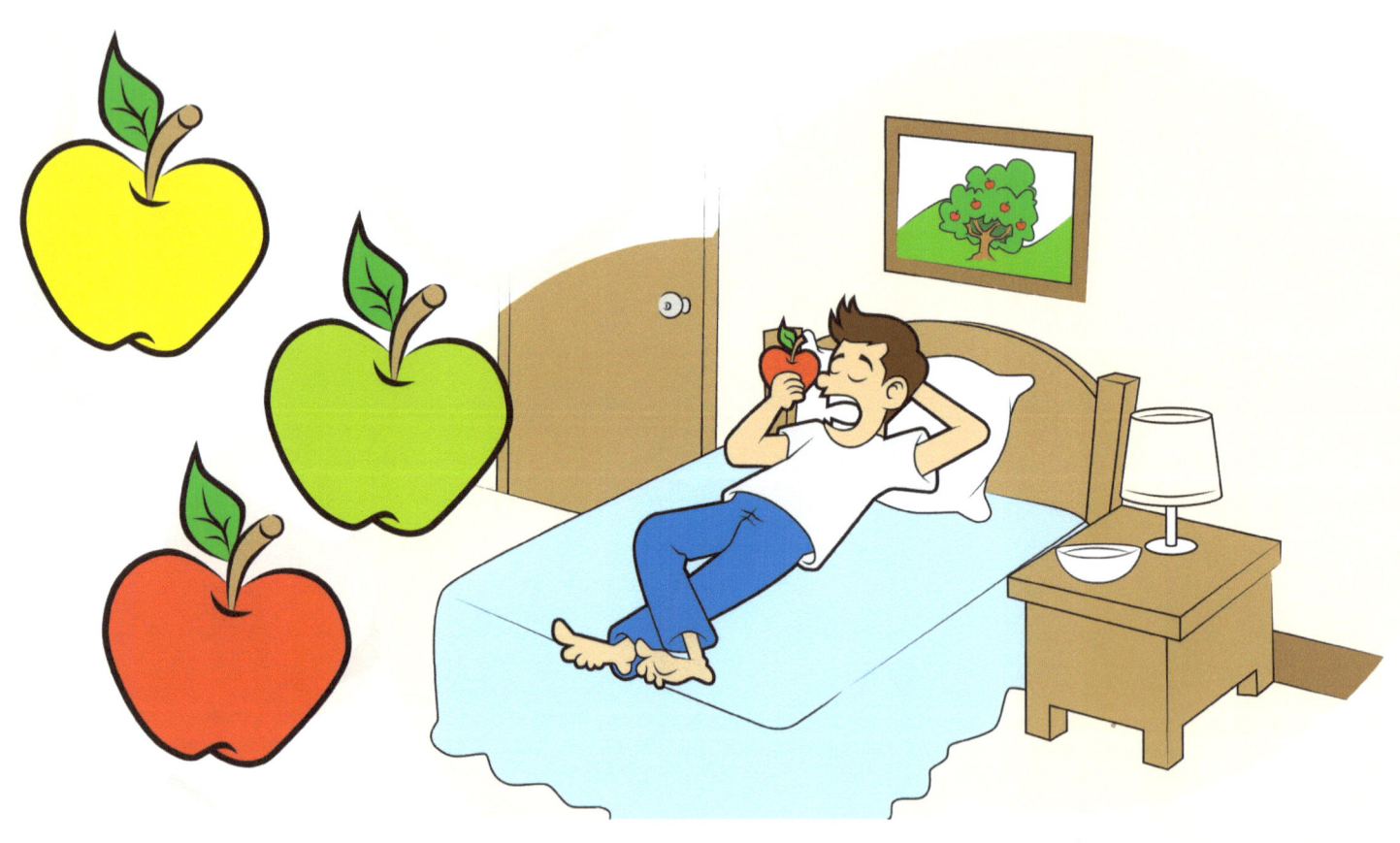

Apples, apples, apples, yellow, green and red.

I'll eat apples anywhere, even on my bed!

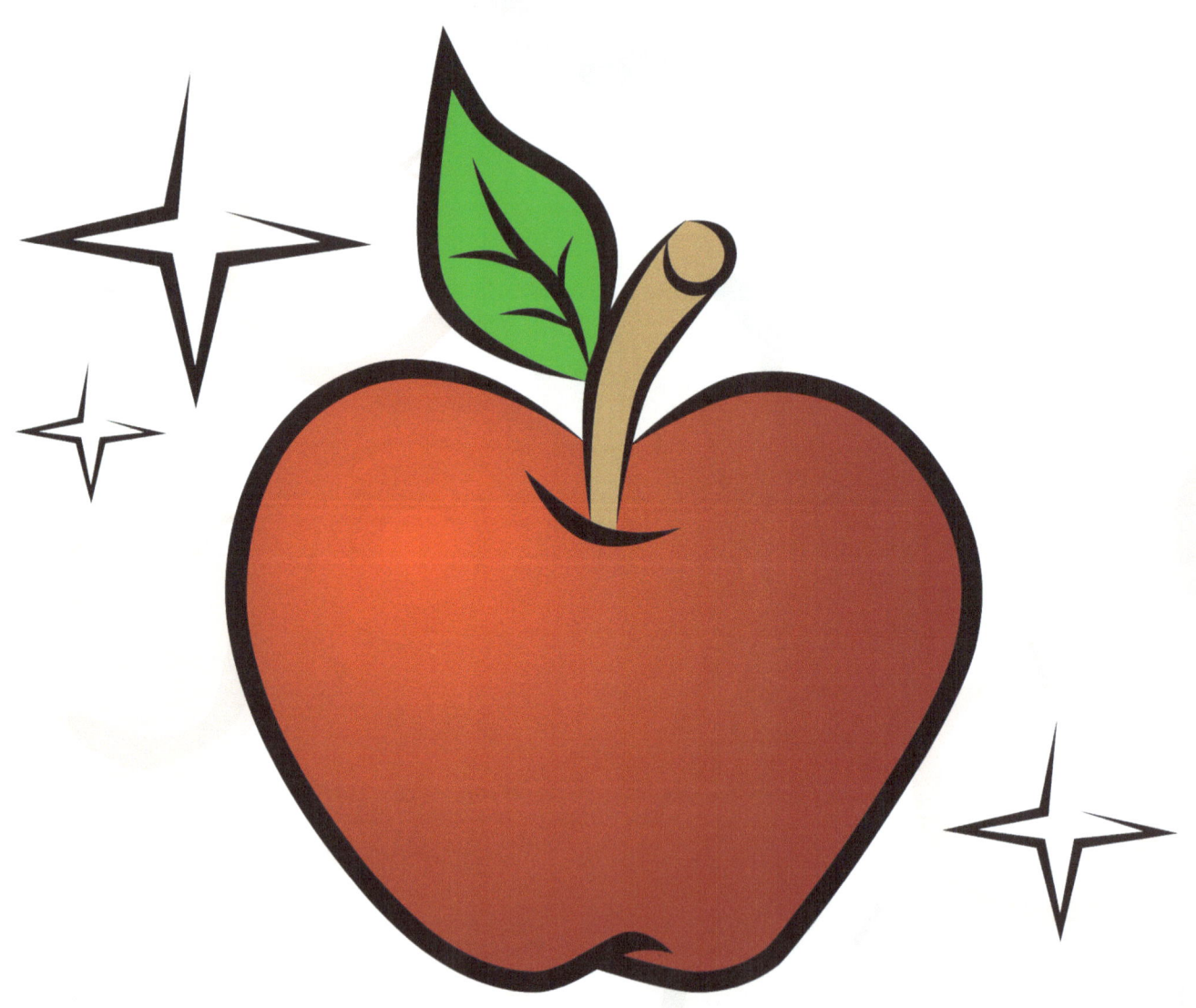

Crisp and juicy, tart and sweet, the perfect snack, the perfect treat.

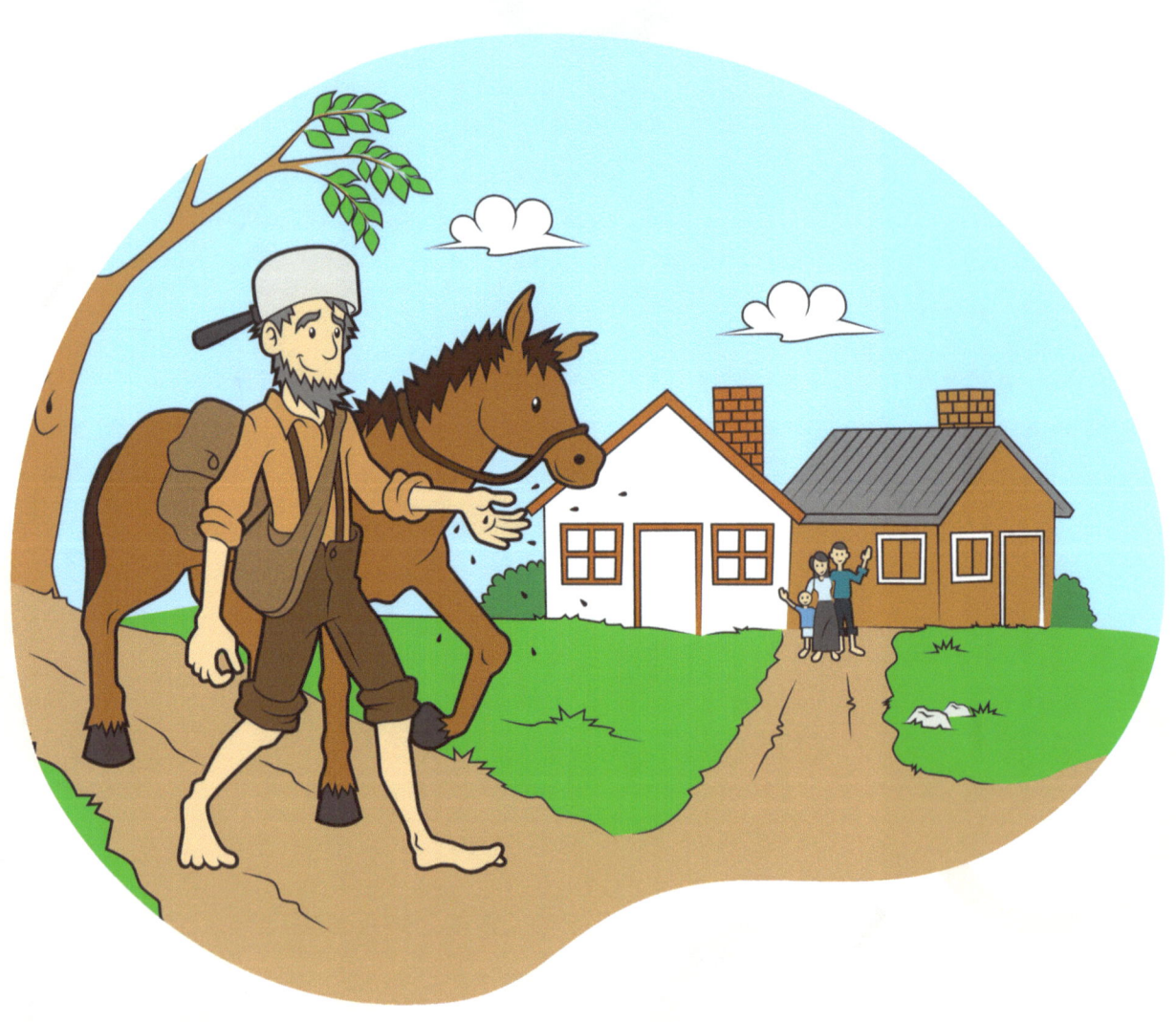

Johnny Appleseed was a man, who traveled far and wide, from home to home he walked each day, a pack horse at his side. He planted seeds and nurtured trees, and charmed the nation with selfless deeds.

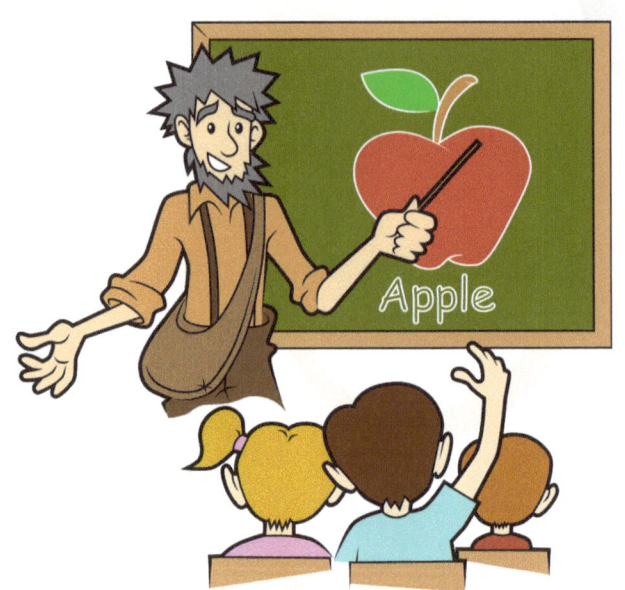

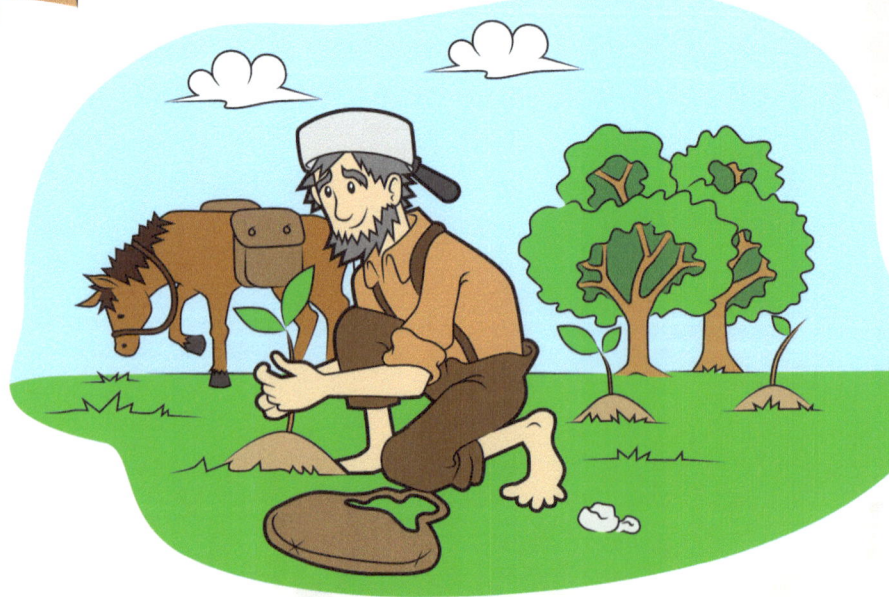

A legacy of orchards, an apple pioneer, a humble caring teacher, mother nature's keeper.

Apple juice, pure and sweet, cures a cough and beats the heat.

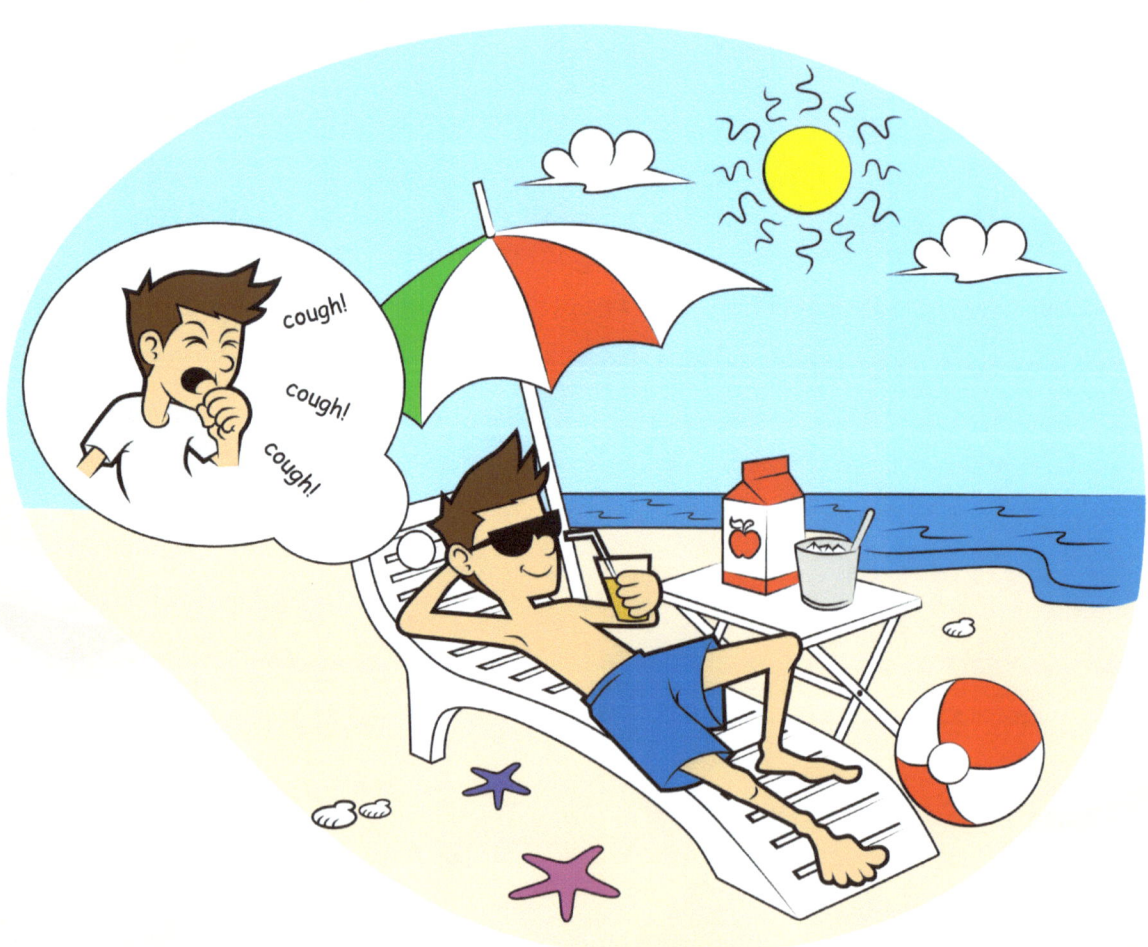

Apple cider, cold and brown, a little bite to turn a frown.

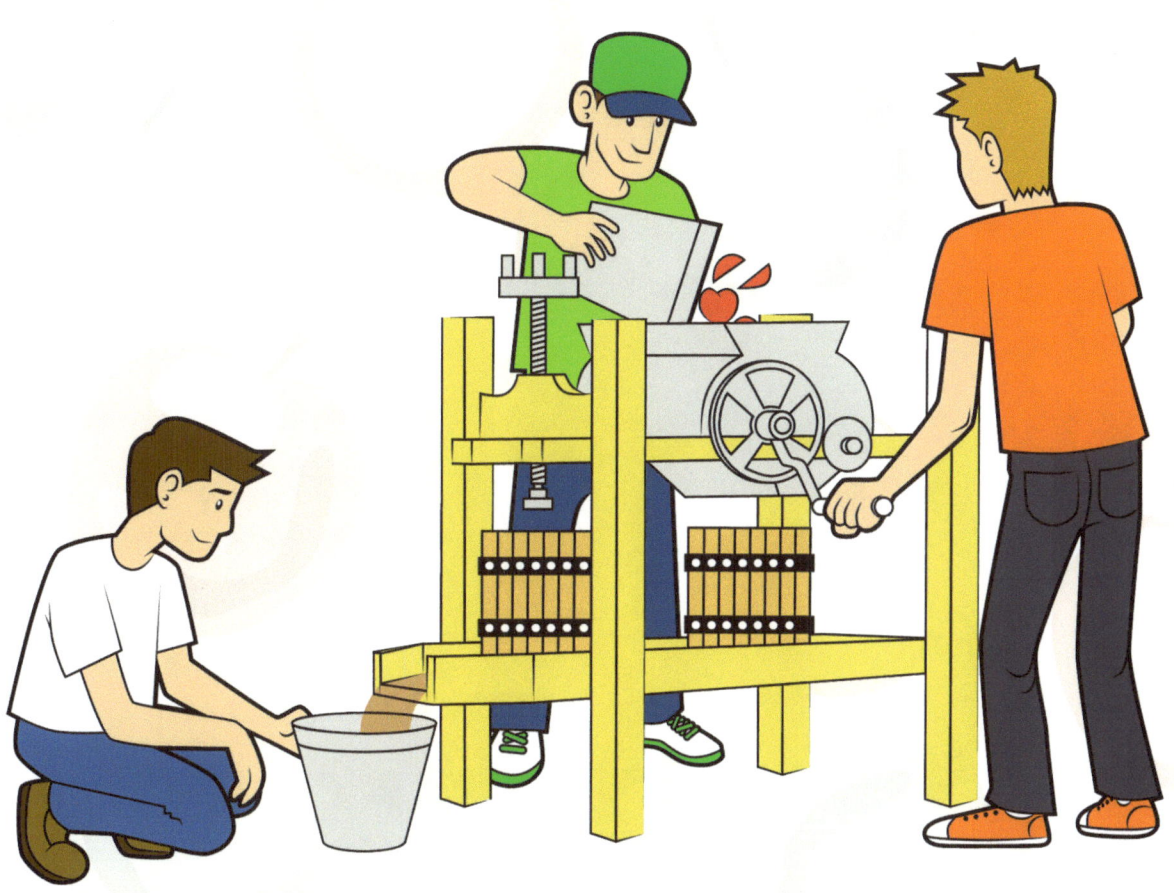

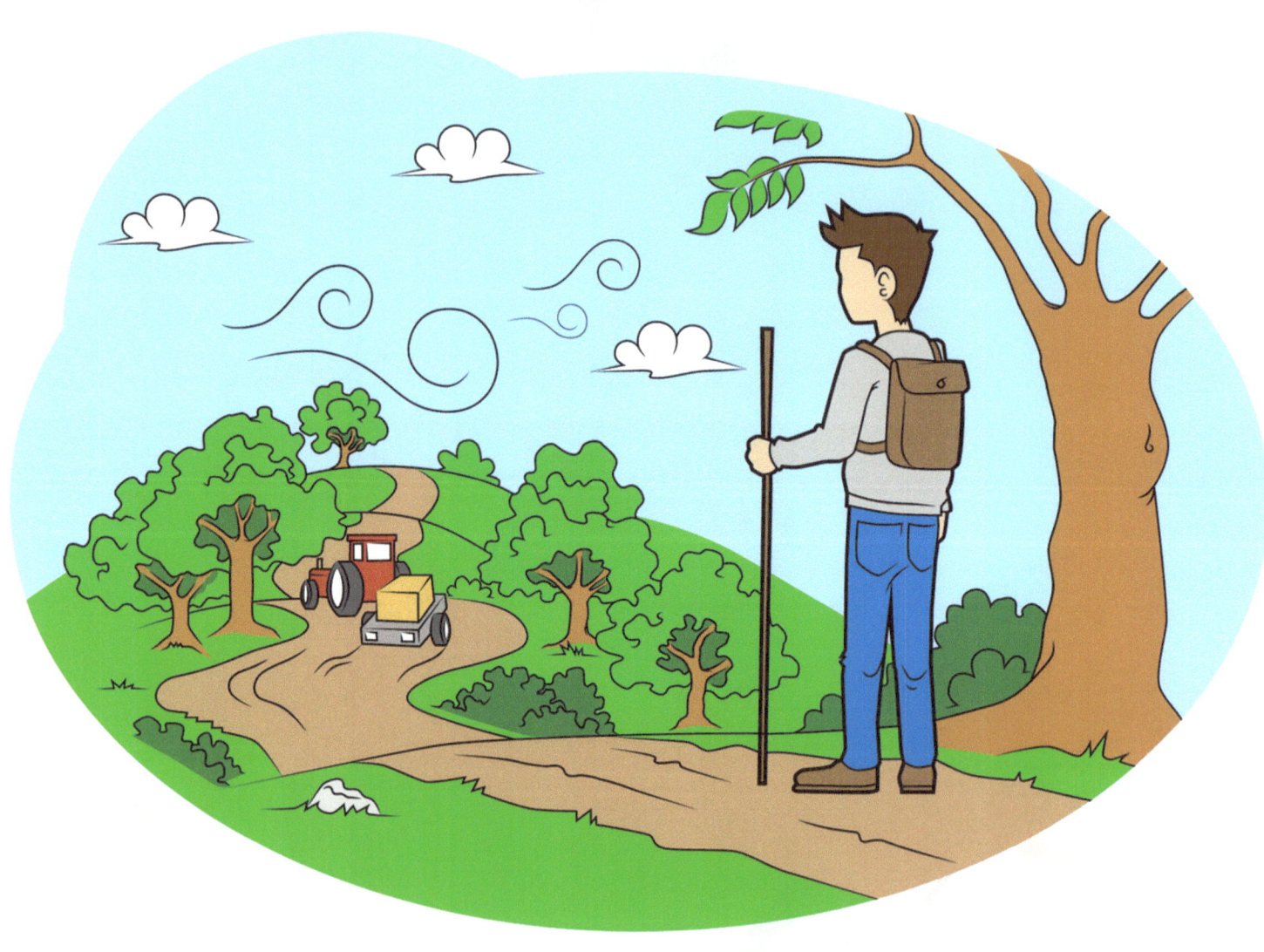

Sneakers worn, jeans with a rip, a cozy sweater, a walking stick. A fall morning, a bright blue sky, a cool breeze blowing, summer's goodbye.

An old steep logging road, muddy from tractors with heavy loads. The green canopy yielding to Autumn gold, the path opens on a field untold.

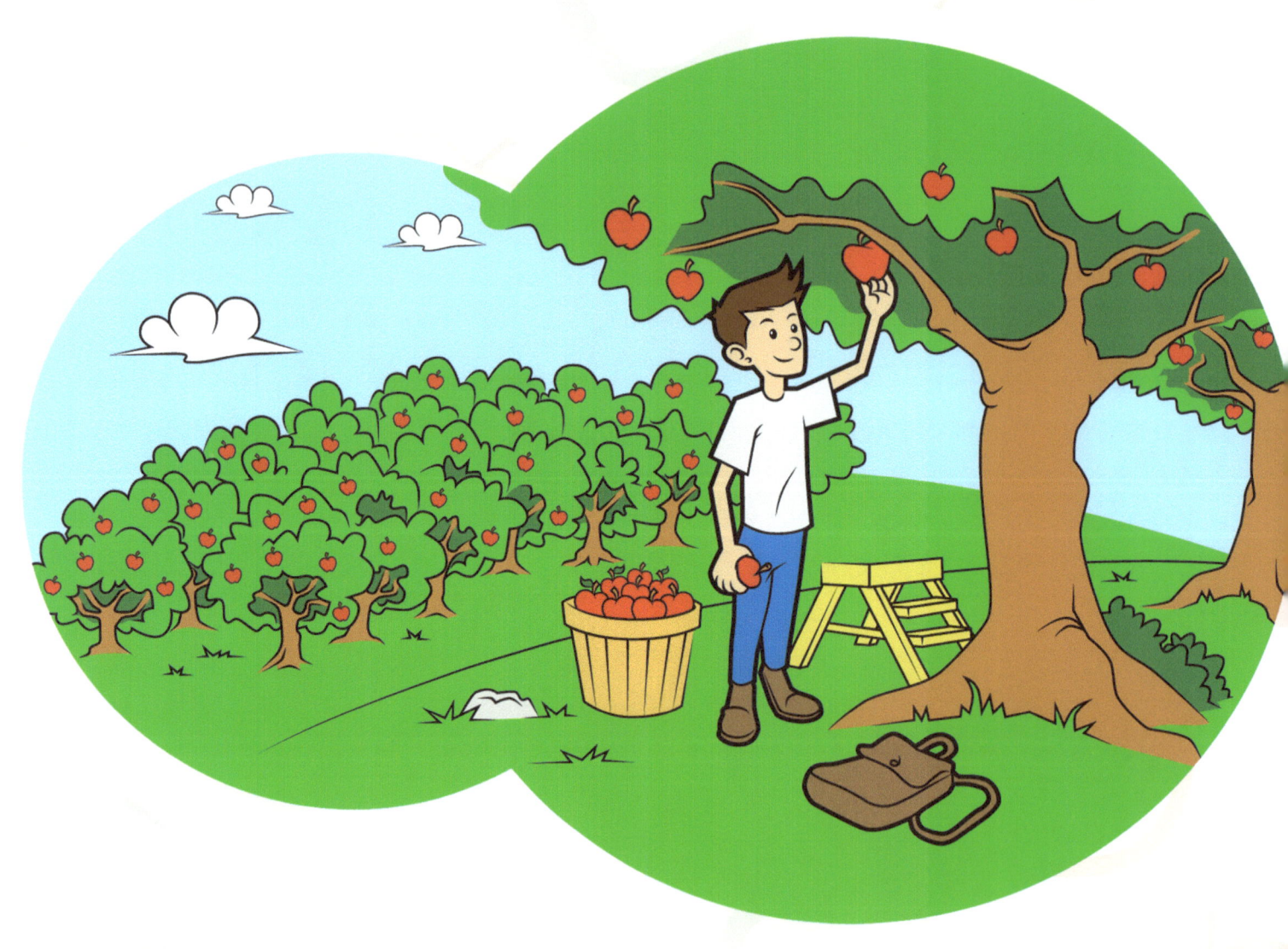

Rows and rows of apple trees, giving trees so splendid, branches bow, leaves rustle, red ornaments suspended.

A day picking apples is time well spent, a day picking apples is heaven sent.

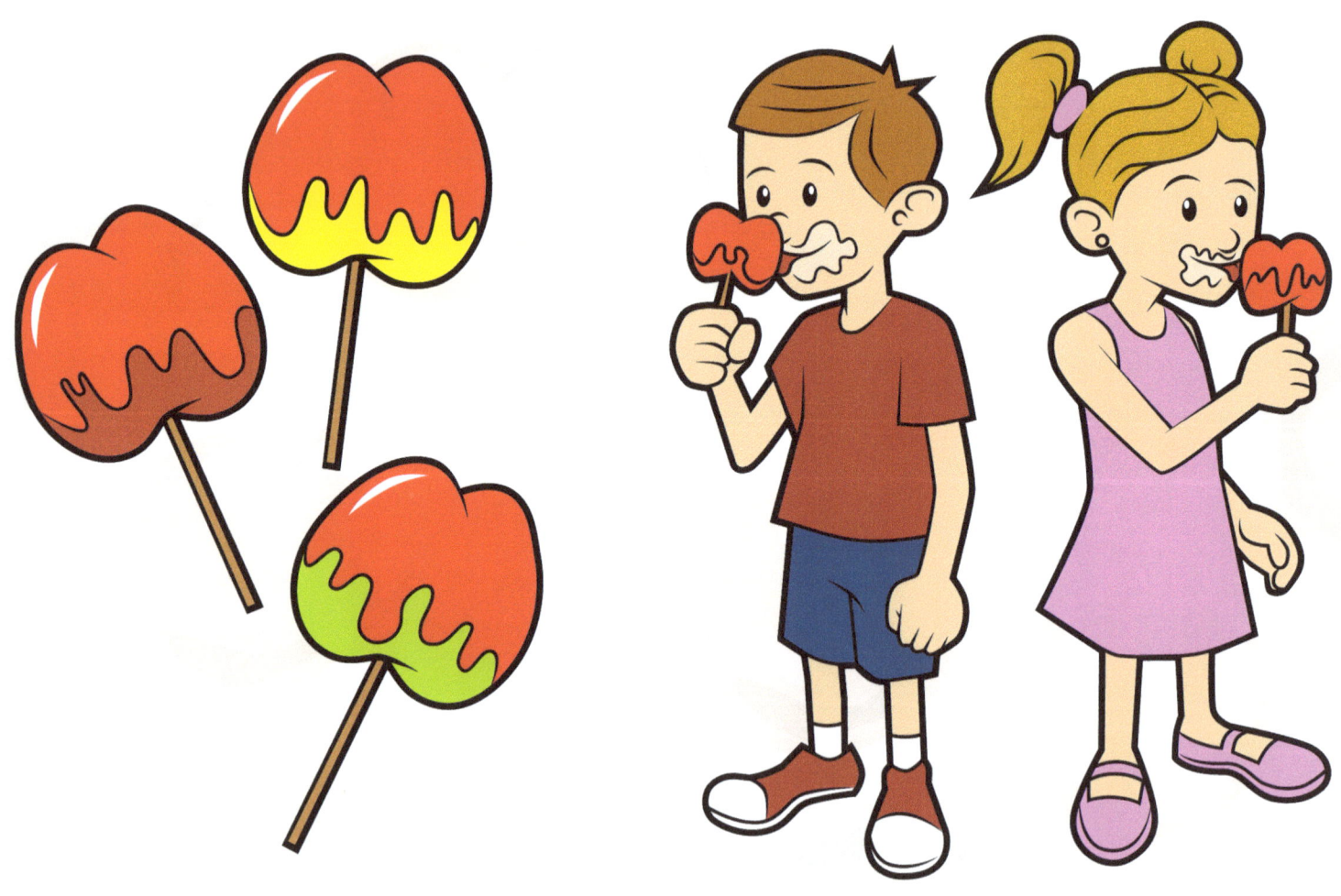

Candied apples on pointy sticks, happy children with frantic licks. Fairground fare without compare, sticky faces everywhere.

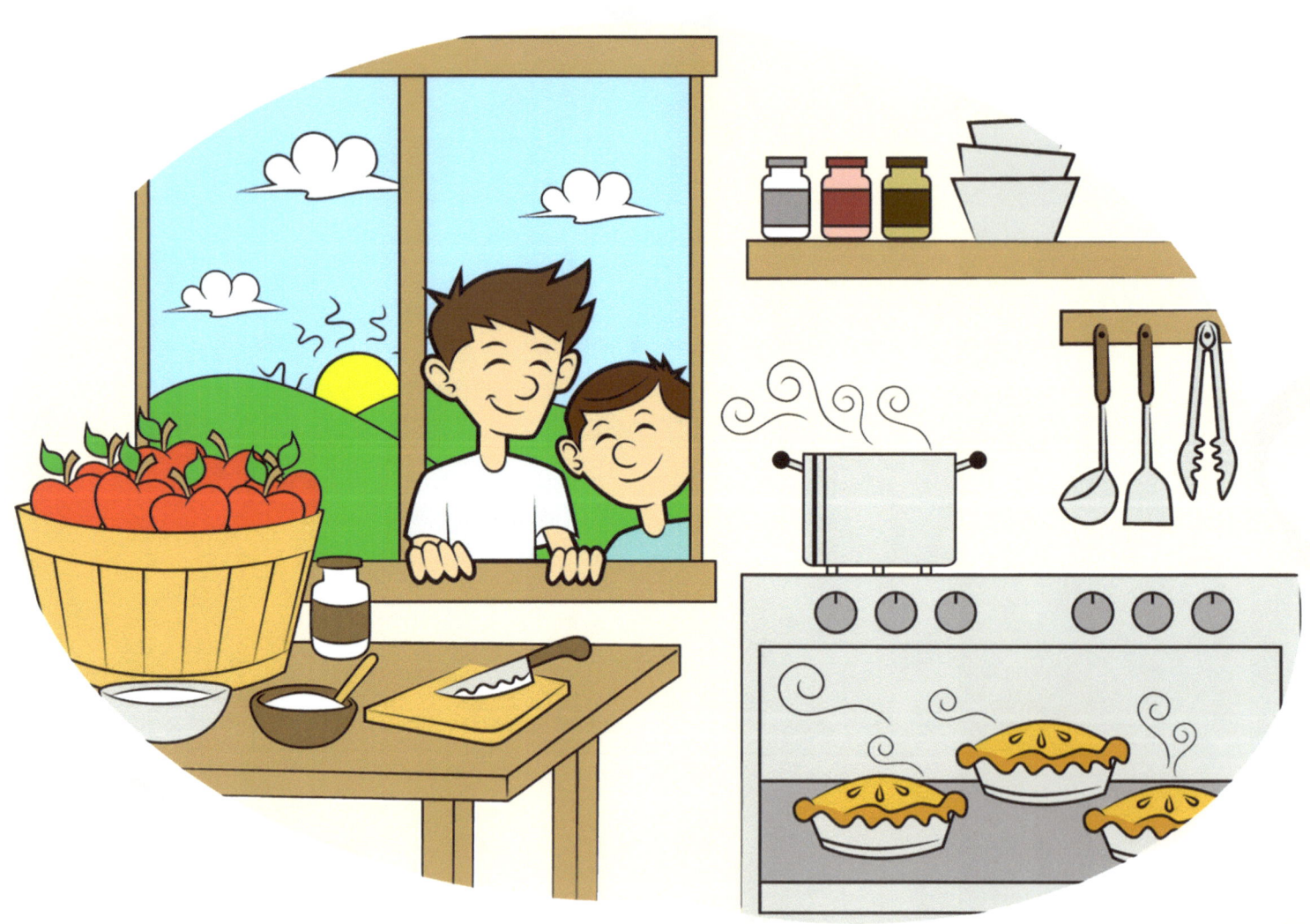

A bushel on her table, the sun fades on the hill, the smells from Grandma's kitchen, draw us to her sill.

She peeled and sliced and baked all day, tireless in the heat, to make a splendid medley, of sweet and tasty treats.

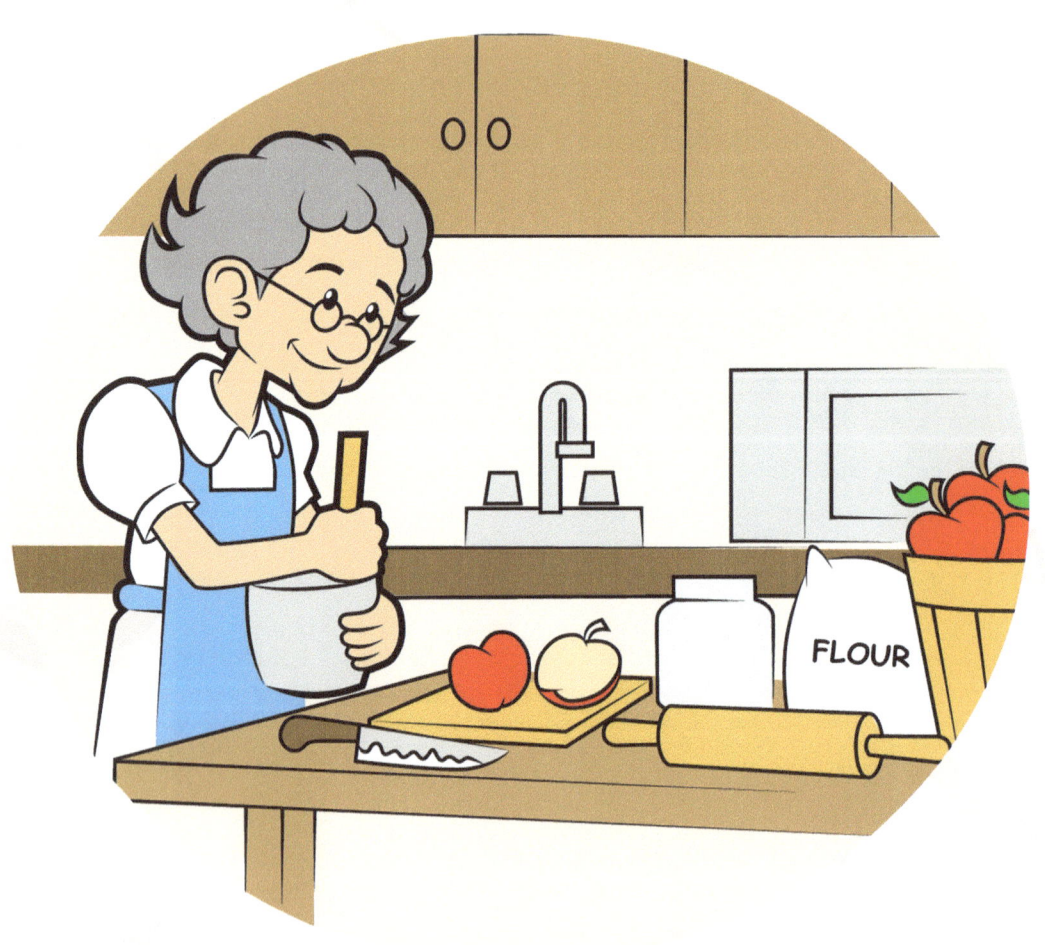

Her apple sauce is the best, a touch of sugar and cinnamon zest. Apple pie, apple crisp, apple strudel, and apple cake. Her delicacies unrivaled, a divinity of flake.

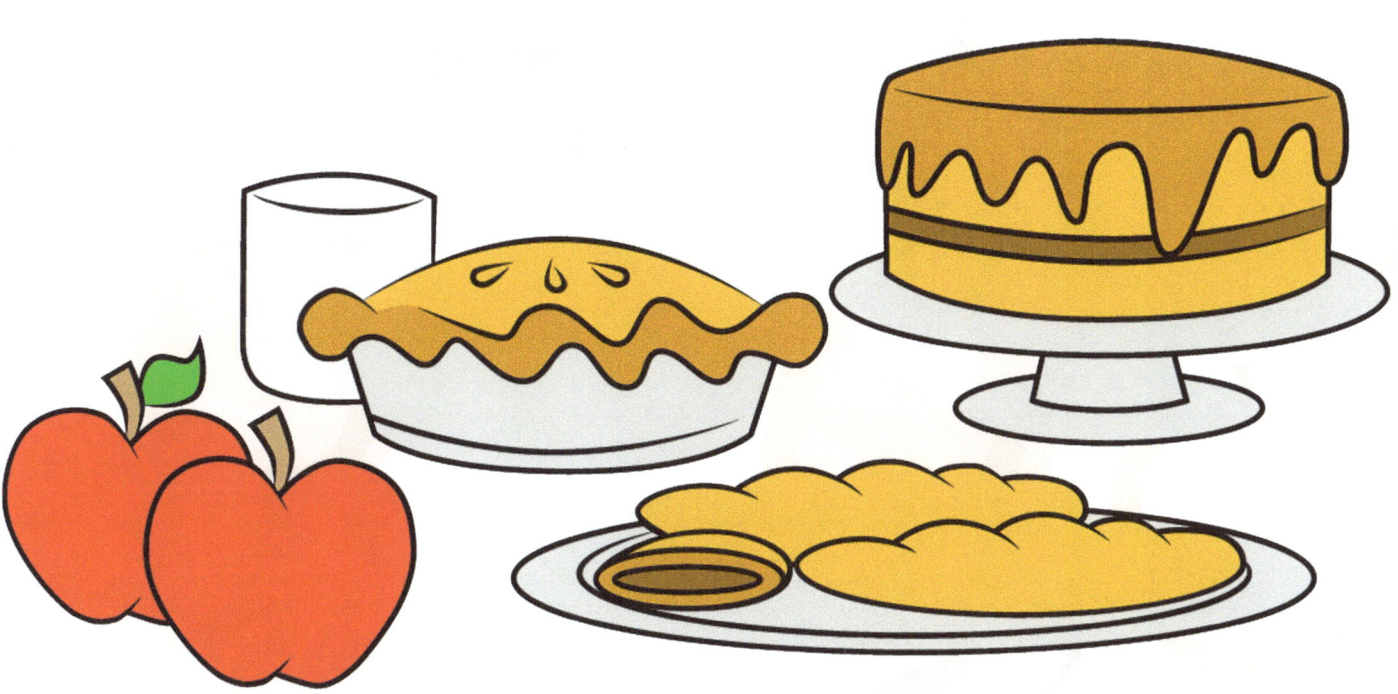

Apples, apples, apples, yellow, green and red.

I'll eat apples anywhere, even on my bed!

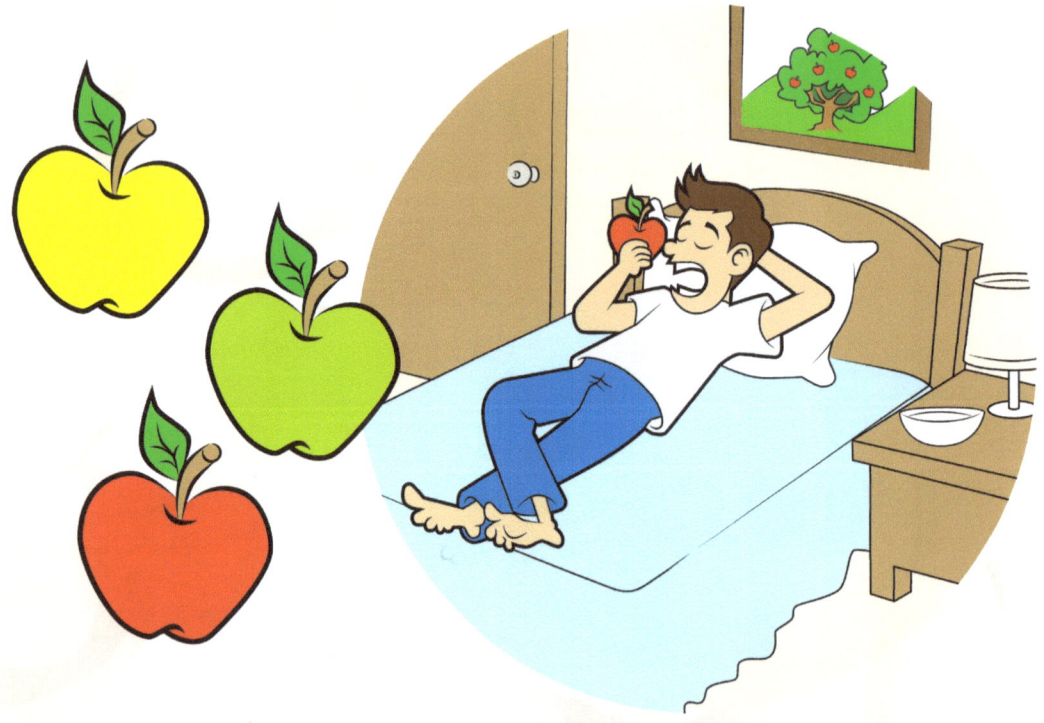

Tim Dailey lives in Littleton, Colorado with his wife and three kids (Joey, Logan and Clara) and their cat, Boots. When not writing poetry about the things he loves, he works at Dailey Partners (www.daileypartners.com), an investment banking firm that assists fast-growing companies in venture capital fund raising and mergers and acquisitions. Tim's favorite hobbies include playing the violin, building snow sculptures, and continuing to add to the 'I Love…' series. Tim hopes that his poems, along with the photographs and illustrations, will offer a moment of joy to every reader. Finally, he wants to thank the talented photographers, illustrators and book designers that have made this series possible. For more books from the 'I Love…' series, please visit: www.timdaileypoems.com.

www.ingramcontent.com/pod-product-compliance
Lightning Source LLC
Chambersburg PA
CBHW060823290526
45792CB00005BB/1769